BIRTH CONTROL
AND
SAFE SEX

Sex Secrets Every Couple

Needs to Know

Dr. Mary Ann Martínez

Marcasa Books

Marcasa Books
PO Box 5442
Caguas, PR 00726

This book contains information that is intended to help the readers be better informed. It is presented as general advice. Always consult your doctor for your individual needs. This book is not intended to be a substitute for the professional advice of a licensed therapist or licensed physician. The reader should consult with their healthcare professional in any matters relating to his/her physical and mental health.

To everyone seeking love.

CONTENTS

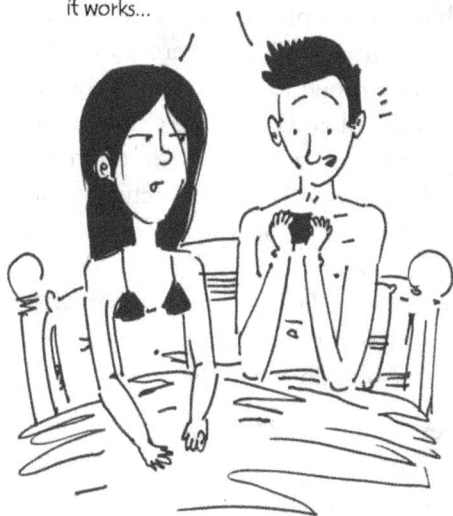

About Birth Control and Safe Sex

The logic is simple!

If you are sexually active and not willing to conceive, birth control is something you need to master at. Whether you are in your teens or older, married or unmarried, a parent or still considering it -- every man and woman who enjoy sex needs to know and understand all there is about this particular topic.

Nothing is simple in this day and age. In more conservative times, children were inevitable in married life. Men and women both restrained themselves before they were married and ready for children, and once they had the license, it wasn't up to them to limit their number of offspring. No one actually thought about birth control back in those days, at least not men and women who already had a family. More than six or seven children in a family were normal, and respectable married women did not think of stopping until they were past their childbearing age.

However, the situation is entirely different these days. Most couples are opting for not more than one or two children, some even none. This is where different methods of birth control come in handy for them, since of course they want to enjoy sex with each other without having to worry about an unwanted pregnancy. Birth control methods and procedures are varied and more common among married couples, as well as couples in a committed relationship with a single partner.

On the other hand, the concept of safe sex is a different matter. People who are sexually active but not limited to a spouse or a single partner are mainly concerned with keeping themselves safe against a number of Sexually Transmitted Diseases (STDs) that are gradually becoming a threat. These diseases are what worry them more than a pregnancy care because most of them can be fatal.

This is where both the concepts of birth control and safe sex overlap, but also differentiates. Both methods prevent a pregnancy, but safe sex can also prevent STDs – which is more important to sexually active people with multiple partners.

Yes, it is easy to get confused about which procedure is better and which less effective, especially if you are on the verge of choosing one. The best decision can be taken only when you are aware of all the facts, and that's what you are going to get in this book. Safe sex and birth control – both concepts have been described here in details, along with all the methods available today.

Trust me, there are more methods available than you can imagine!

This book is for everyone! From teenagers who are curious but cautious, to men and women who enjoy their freedom, from couples who are physically intimate but not ready for children, to couples who have had enough children already. Knowledge is power and you will find a good stock of knowledge here in this book.

Knowing everything there is about the correct procedures of birth control and safe sex can save you from an unwanted pregnancy, heartache and even a serious disease. So go on, start reading! Know all your facts before you decide on something. Because, as the eternal truth warns us about:

"Prevention is better than cure!"

Common and Effective Birth Control Methods

The name is pretty self-explanatory. By using "birth control" methods, you are preventing a "birth"; or more accurately, a conception. The most common reason for using birth control methods is to stop a pregnancy from occurring, which could be both when you are not ready for a baby or when you already have the required number of children you want.

Birth control methods are therefore more common in families where a couple is married or in a committed relationship with each other. This is because birth control measures mainly prevent pregnancies; they almost never give protection against Sexually Transmitted Diseases. Most of these diseases spread when a person is sexually active with more than one partner at a time.

According to the data[1] collected in October 2012 for the Center for Disease Control, U.S. Department of Health and Human Services,[2] 77% of the total population of married women of childbearing age always uses birth control methods to prevent conception. Reasonably, 44% of women who have never married use birth control procedures as they are less sexually active than women who are married. According to the same study, at present more than 62% of the total female population in the United States of America who are at risk of pregnancy – i.e. of childbearing age and sexually active – use one or more methods of contraception.

On the other hand, the number of women from ages 15 to 44 who have never used birth control measures in their life is less than 1%.[3]

When it comes to birth control measures, other factors - such as religion, race or background – does not make a big difference to the numbers. This is evident from a number of studies conducted on this topic, particularly the paper published in 2011 titled "Countering Conventional Wisdom: New Evidence Religion and Contraceptive Use"[4] by R.K. Jones and J. Dreweke. In U.S.A., 89% of women who are Catholics and 90% women who are Protestants regularly use contraceptive methods and are currently using at least one method.

Among them, 83% women are black, 91% are from Hispanic origin, 91% are white and 90% with an Asian background in the United States who are currently using birth control methods to prevent pregnancy.

Socially, the responsibility of birth control falls mostly on the female partner in a relationship with the exception of a condom – which is a male oriented birth control measure, and a vasectomy. This is because it is the sexually active women who get pregnant, not the man.

Also, for this same reason, birth control measures are only necessary in traditional relationships between a man and a woman, rather than in same-sex relationships and marriages. In homosexual relationships between two men or two women, birth control is not necessary because conception is not possible. Safe sex, yes – but that's a completely different topic that needs further discussion!

Choosing the Right Birth Control Method

There are a number of methods to choose from if your main concern is to prevent a pregnancy, but you need to choose the one that suits your lifestyle and health more.

- If you are looking for a permanent solution, i.e. so that you will never be able to conceive, two solutions are vasectomy for men and tubal ligation for women. Not many people opt for these procedures as they are irreversible and it is always desirable to have an option.
- If not permanent, there are a few long-term but reversible techniques, i.e. an implant or Intra-Uterine Device (IUD) for women.
- Hormonal contraception, which includes contraceptive pills, injections and rings.
- Both male and female barrier methods, i.e. condoms for the men and diaphragms for women.
- Emergency Contraceptive Pills for after sexual intercourse without protection.
- Fertility Awareness, i.e. being aware of your (in women) fertile period and having intercourse accordingly.

- Withdrawal method for men so that risk of conception can be avoided.

Of all these methods, the most popular two are undoubtedly the use of condoms for men and the consumption of contraceptive pill for women. Of all these methods, only the use of a male condom can prevent Sexually Transmitted Diseases (STD) or Infection (STI).

Permanent Solutions: Vasectomy & Tubal Ligation

Vasectomy for men and tubal ligation for women - also known as sterilization, are two very serious and completely irreversible birth control procedures. Once performed, it will not be possible for the man or the woman to conceive ever again. Any couple who has the chance or the desire, however remote, to have children in the future, should NEVER consider this option!

Vasectomy

A vasectomy is sterilization in a man, where the tubes that carry sperms from the testicles outside the body are closed forever. When the sperms produced inside the man's body cannot be expelled outside during intercourse, the risks of pregnancy stops completely. The sperms are absorbed by the body instead of being ejaculated with semen. It is only the semen that will be ejaculated which, without the sperm present, cannot contribute to a pregnancy.

There are two ways of performing a vasectomy: *incision method and non-incision method.* An incision method, which takes around 20 minutes, is a method where a miniature incision is made on a man's scrotum to block the tubes with a surgical clip. On the other hand, in a non-incision method, a tiny puncture is made instead of a cut to insert the clip. This method is easier and does not leave a mark, and lessens the chances of bleeding.

Side Effects:

- As mentioned before, this is an irreversible procedure. Even if the surgery can be reversed, it may not be effective and a future pregnancy is impossible.

- A vasectomy is not immediately effective after the procedure. It may take as long as 3 months and more than 15 ejaculations to completely get rid of the sperms those are present beyond the blocks to leave the body. For these three months, ejaculation into a condom or masturbation is recommended before intercourse without protection.

- This procedure does not, in any way, effect masculinity or the desire for intercourse. However, some men have reported trouble in getting satisfaction in intercourse after a vasectomy, mainly due to psychological reasons.

A vasectomy is a 100% effective procedure that prevents the chance of any future conception for a man. However, the decision for a vasectomy should only be taken if you are completely sure that you don't want any biological children in the future, because this procedure cannot be reversed once performed.

Tubal Ligation or Female Sterilization

A tubal ligation – or, tubal sterilization or having your tubes tied – for women is what vasectomy is for men. It is a permanent procedure to ensure that a sexually active woman does not get pregnant even when she doesn't use any protection. This is a simple surgery that can be performed any time, and is usually requested by the patient with a C-Section birth if she wants no more children. The risks are minimum, and the procedure doesn't disturb a woman's menstrual system or her sexual desires.

A tubal ligation can be reversed with another major surgery but is almost never effective. This is why decision for a sterilization surgery should be taken with care. Once performed, this surgery means the woman in question can never get pregnant and have a biological child.

The process of a tubal ligation is simple enough. A small cut is made in the abdomen and the fallopian tubes are blocked off so that the sperms from your partner cannot meet the egg produced in your ovaries. This is another 100% effective way of ensuring that you won't get pregnant in the future. In the first year, the chances of getting pregnant accidently are 1 in 1000, or lower than that.

Side Effects:

- Regret is one of the most common side effects of a tubal ligation. Women who decide to have this surgery in their early 30s may regret their choice later when they are in their 40s and want another child. However, even if reversed, the chances of getting pregnant – especially in their 40s – are hard for a woman.
- A tubal ligation is expensive, but reversing it is costlier.
- Although rare, a sterilization surgery can lead to injury and further complication to the arteries, bowel and bladder.
- In the rare case that a woman can get pregnant after a tubal ligation, it can be an ectopic pregnancy – i.e. when the fertilized egg implants in another part of the abdomen instead

of the uterus. An ectopic pregnancy usually ends in heartbreak and can also be fatal.

Just like vasectomy, it is important that you are completely sure before requesting your gynecologist for a tubal ligation. Once performed, it is near to impossible to get pregnant again and have a biological child.

Long-term Solutions: Implant & IUD

Both of these solutions are for women and can prevent pregnancy for up to 5 years. They have little or no side effects but are more than 99.8% effective, inexpensive and recommended by physicians. Moreover, both implants and Intra-Uterine Devices (IUD) are reversible and can be removed at any time if you want to conceive.

Implant

A birth control implant is a 1.5 inch-long soft rod, something like a match stick that the doctor can insert under the skin of your arm. The stick will slowly produce a hormone named progesterone which will spread around in your body. Progesterone is a special hormone that stops your ovaries from releasing eggs, making it impossible for you to get pregnant. At the same time, progesterone makes your cervical mucus thicker than normal, and unable to receive sperms after intercourse.

The dual effect of progesterone in your body makes this method almost 99.95% effective with very few chances of unintentional pregnancy. A single implant can work for about 3 years and can be removed at any time. Once removed, pregnancy can be immediate with no side effects.

Besides, an implant is completely invisible under your skin which helps if you want to keep your birth control measure private.

Side Effects:

- For some women, period can become irregular - lighter and fewer; for others, heavier.

- Almost everyone experiences light spotting and cramping between periods for the first 6 to 12 months of implantation.

- For some woman, period can stop altogether after the first year of light spotting.

- Other common symptoms include light nausea, sore breasts, slight weight gain and headache.

The side effects of implantation are somewhat similar to symptoms of pregnancy, but there's nothing to be worried about if these indications are seen. With an implant, the chances of conception are almost slim.

Intra-Uterine Device (IUD)

An IUD is a small, T-shaped device that is inserted directly into a woman's uterus to prevent a conception. Based on your need, an IUD can prevent pregnancy from 3 to 12 years.

An Intra-Uterine Device can be of two types – copper or hormonal. The IUD made from copper stops the sperms from meeting the eggs and can be effective for about 12 years. On the other hand, the hormonal IUD works like an implant by making the cervical mucus thicker than normal, preventing pregnancies. There are different brands of hormonal IUDs that are effective against conception for 3 and 5 years.

IUDs are extremely safe for most women; however, if you have or ever had cervical or uterus cancer that went untreated, this method is not for you. Women who are already pregnant should not insert an IUD into their uterus; neither should women who have had a history of Sexually Transmitted Infections (STI) in the past. Other than that, any woman who is sexually active and doesn't want children in the near future can safely use IUDs to prevent unintentional pregnancies.

The perfect time to insert an IUD would be in the middle of a menstrual cycle, when the cervix is already open. Besides, many women opt for a long-term measure like IUD after childbirth or an abortion. The procedure is easy and starts working within a week of insertion. For the first week, a secondary method is recommended.

Removal is also an easy process but should always be done by a professional. In some rare cases, a simple surgery may be needed for removal, especially if the IUD has been left inside for many years. Under any circumstances, it shouldn't be removed by anyone other than a doctor or a professional using special surgical tool.

Side Effects:

- With a copper IUD, period may get heavier and cramps may increase.
- With hormonal IUD, periods may become irregular the first 6 months.
- For the first 3-6 months of insertion, light spotting can be seen.
- Immediately after insertion, a little pain can be experienced in the abdomen area.

- Cramping will be present for the first week in most women.

This method is almost painless and more than 99% effective. Although there are a few side effects, as mentioned above, it is one of the most popular and common methods used by women to enjoy a spontaneous sex life with no worries about getting pregnant. Conception can be possible immediately after removal, and can be done at any time.

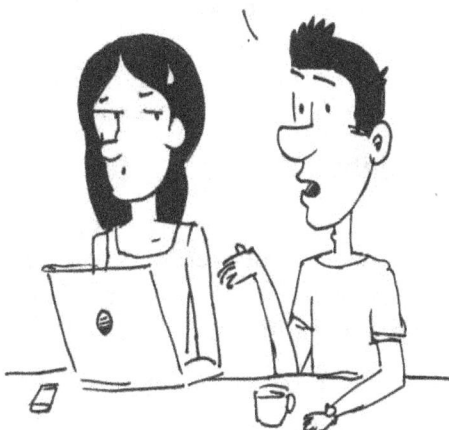

Hormonal Contraception: Pills, Injections, Patches and Rings

Hormonal contraceptive measures are also for women who want neither a long-term solution nor the risk of conception. These measures introduce chemically produced hormones into a woman's body, in the forms of contraceptive pills, injections, rings or patches. These artificially introduced hormones temporarily changes the female reproductive system in a number of ways – by thickening the cervical mucus, lining the walls of the uterus, slowing down male sperm and by reducing the ability of the fertilized egg so that the woman cannot conceive.

Contraceptive Pills

Contraceptive pills have been a popular choice of birth control by women all over the world for a number of years, especially before the advent of other short-term options like a diaphragm or female condoms.

Available in a number of international and local brands throughout the world, these are miniature pills that contain two synthetic hormones named estrogen and progestin. These two hormones prevent an egg from leaving the ovaries, which stops conception by not meeting male sperms. As with other methods of birth control, the extra hormone in the body also makes the cervical mucus thicker, making it a problem for the egg to join the sperms.

Mainly two types of contraceptive pills are available in the market under different brands: *combination pills* and *progestin-only 'mini' pills*. Combination pills contain both progestin and estrogen and help prevent conception by suppressing the body's ovulation every month. Each month's supply of combination pill includes 3 week's worth of hormonal pills as well as one week's worth of placebo pills that will regulate your period.

Mini pills, on the other hand, only contain progestin and are prescribed to women who have severe reaction to combination pills. These pills only prevent pregnancy but do not regulate menstrual cycles.

Both of these pills need to be swallowed with water every day, at exactly the same time for them to work properly. If the pills for two consecutive days are forgotten, the cycle breaks and has to be started again from the next period. For the rest of the month, secondary birth control is recommended. Otherwise, the chance of pregnancy is always there for women who are sexually active.

Side Effects:

- It is possible that you may have some severe reactions to a particular brand of contraceptive pills. If that happens, the easy solution would be to switch to another brand after the next menstrual cycle.

- While combination pills usually regulate period, it is also possible for you to miss your period for many months altogether. Switching your brand may help, but there's nothing to be worried about with irregular periods.

- Combination pills can be troublesome to women who are 35 years and older *and* smokers; for them, progestin-only pills are prescribed.

- Some common side effects of contraceptive pills include nausea and headaches, soreness in your breasts, slight spotting between periods. All these side effects do not happen to the same woman and they are not severe or serious.

- Although there are no scientific facts that support the idea, many women have complained of weight gain after regularly taking birth control pills. It is possible to experience some fluid retention in the hip and breast areas with these pills, which can add to your weight.

Women, who have a history of heart diseases in their family or are obese, should look for other methods of birth control as contraceptive pills can increase risk for clotting of blood. Also, these pills are not recommended for women who have a history of breast cancer, high blood pressure that cannot be controlled or severe migraine.

Other than that, contraceptive pills are one of the most effective methods and widely popular for birth control. The effectiveness rates of these pills are 99.9%, which means that 1 in 100 women might get pregnant in the first year of taking pills; the risk decreases even further after continuous use for many years.

Contraceptive Injection

This is a special shot named Depo-Provera that can prevent pregnancy for up to 3 months for a woman of childbearing age who is also sexually active.

These shots are given on the arms or the buttocks every 3 months if you are looking for short-term birth control measures. As with other hormonal methods, these injections introduce the progestin hormone into the body which stops the eggs from leaving the ovaries to meet the sperms released from your male partner's body. At the same time, this hormone thickens the cervical mucus and keeps the sperms away from the egg, thus preventing conception.

Side Effects:

Contraceptive injections come with a number of side effects on the first few months that eventually goes away over time, including:

- Soreness in breasts
- Irregular periods
- Unnatural weight gain
- Change of appetite
- Mood swings and depression
- Vaginal Irritation
- Severe headache similar to migraine pains
- Nausea and dizziness
- Hair loss/increased hair
- Loss of sexual desire

In fact, some of the symptoms can be mistaken for a pregnancy scare, especially a missed period, change of appetite, headaches and mood swings. However, these side effects fade and eventually disappear within a few months.

Contraceptive injections are about 94% effective and a painless way to stay worry-free for 3 months at a time. If you decide to have children, miss a shot and conception can be almost immediate.

Contraceptive Patches

Contraceptive Patches are Band Aid-like square patches that are beige in color and made of plastic. They can be attached to the skin like a Band-Aid and the hormones from the patch are soaked through the skin to your body. The patches contain progestin hormones that work to suppress ovulation and prevent pregnancy.

These patches can be attached almost anywhere on the body, i.e. arms, legs, buttocks, hips, back, stomach, etc; they should not be attached near a sensitive part of the body including breasts or lower abdomen, though. They need to be changed every week and you won't have a period on the weeks you are wearing a patch. If you want your period to be regular, just stop wearing a patch on the fourth week after three weeks of using. Your scheduled period will come once you've removed the patch.

It makes the procedure simple if you designate a special day of the week as your "patch changing day", like Saturday. If you've attached your first patch on a Saturday, do it again the next Saturday until you want to regulate your period or get pregnant. For the next cycle, put on your patch within five days of your period. This way, you can be safe again from unintentional pregnancy almost immediately.

This is one of the easiest methods of birth control, just like sticking a Band-Aid on a cut, a painless method that is 91% to 99.7% effective.

Side Effects:

- Skin irritation is a common side effect of these patches, quite understandably.
- These patches are less effective on obese women who weigh over 198 pounds (90 kg) and over.
- Spotting and light bleeding between periods, nausea and lightheadedness and sore breasts are common symptoms of contraceptive patches, but they lessen over time.

On the bright side, these patches are known to help clean up acne caused by hormonal reasons. If used correctly, they are effective and an easy method of preventing pregnancies, one that many women choose.

Vaginal Rings

These are small and soft plastic rings that are 5.5cm in diameter and 4mm thick. They need to be folded and inserted into the vagina where they release the progestin hormone to suppress ovulation and stop pregnancy for 3 weeks straight. At the beginning of the fourth week, these rings need to be removed and thrown away for regular period to start. After 7 days of not wearing one, a new vaginal ring needs to be inserted for the next cycle.

Neither partner will be able to feel the presence of the ring inside the vagina during intercourse. Placing a ring in the vagina will not, in any way, disturb sex with a partner, and there is very little chance of it being dislodged. If inserted and used correctly, a vaginal ring can be up to 99% effective to stop conception.

Side Effects:

- The side effects of vaginal rings are similar to those of other hormonal methods, ranging from light to severe headaches, more vaginal discharge, nausea and dizziness.
- Some women may experience reduced bleeding and less painful cramps during their period.
- Very rarely, some women develop a case of thrombosis, which is a kind of blood clot that is treatable.
- Sometimes, not often, the ring may fall off. If something like that happens, it is possible to wash it with warm water and insert it again for the rest of the cycle. Or, you can wait for

the cycle to end to insert a new one. In this case, secondary birth control methods should be used.

Both insertion and removal of vaginal rings is easy and painless. If you experience pain or bleeding, which is rare but possible, it is important to notify your doctor immediately.

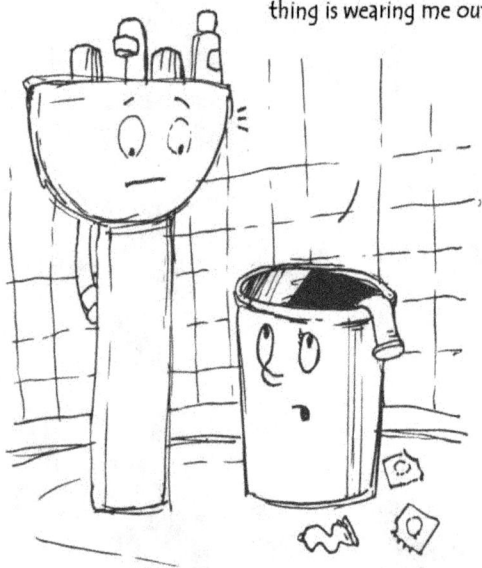

Barrier Method: Diaphragm, Cap, Sponge and Condoms

Many women who are looking for effective birth control methods aren't too enthusiastic with hormonal methods. This is either because they prefer not to experiment with their hormones or because these methods don't suit their body. For these women who aren't too comfortable with hormonal methods or long-term arrangements, the perfect solution lies in barrier method.

Among barrier methods, the use of male condom is most common and widely adopted. There are a few equally effective methods similar to use of condoms, i.e. diaphragms, cervical cap and sponge and spermicide.

Diaphragms

Diaphragms are small and thin and made from soft silicon, resembling a dome; they need to be inserted into a woman's vagina and rests just above the cervix during sexual intercourse. This is a temporary solution of birth control; a diaphragm doesn't have to be kept inside the vagina at all times, but inserted at least two hours before sex. When used correctly, they are 86% to 94% effective to prevent conception.

The first fitting needs to be done under the guidance of a gynecologist or your physician. The largest diaphragm that fits the opening of your cervix needs to be chosen with the help of a professional. There are a few options to choose from, although the activities are the same: *a flat one, a coil of a spring diaphragm.*

Diaphragms are great for women who are sexually active but not very regular. Unfortunately, the use of a diaphragm rules out the chance of spontaneous sex, since it needs to be inserted a few hours before the anticipation of sexual intercourse.

Every time you insert a diaphragm into your cervix, it needs to be filled with spermicide – which is a variety of creams and lotions that destroy sperms. The sperms from your male partner will be stopped by the spermicide in your diaphragm and prevent any chance of conception. One application of spermicide lasts about two hours, so if you have inserted your diaphragm earlier than two hours, an additional application of spermicide may be needed before sex.

After sex, the diaphragm needs to be kept inside for six to eight hours to make sure all the sperms are gone. After removing – which is easy using your fingers – it needs to be cleaned with warm water and a mild soap, and kept separately in its case away from harmful chemicals. Holes or cracks in your diaphragm will increase the chances of pregnancy; therefore, after each use, it is important to check your diaphragm. You can do it by holding it under a bright light or filling it with water.

Side Effects:

- Diaphragms have a tendency to dislodge sometimes, which can be problematic for unprotected sex. In case that happens, emergency contraception pills need to be taken.
- Weight gain or loss can lead to changes in the way diaphragms are fitted inside your

vagina, as change in weight can lead to change in the size of the opening of your cervix.

• After pregnancy and childbirth, the opening of the cervix increases manifold in size; this can require the refitting of your diaphragm.

• In many cases, diaphragms can cause irritation and discomfort – both in the vagina of the woman and the penis of the man.

• Bladder infection and unusual amount of vaginal discharge are also common side effects of diaphragms.

Diaphragms are small and compact, and can be carried around with you on your adventures. With regular practice, it is easy to insert and remove, as well as to care for. The day you decide to get pregnant, you won't have to do anything other than stop using your diaphragms. More importantly, they don't affect your periods in any way!

Cervical Caps

A Cervical cap or a cervical cover works in the same way as a diaphragm, placed inside the vagina at the opening of the cervix. These caps look like a cup and are held at the cervix with suction, unlike a diaphragm which is fitted around the muscles of the vagina.

Cervical caps are also 84% to 91% effective; however, for women who have already given birth, the rate decreases to 68%-74%. This is because the opening of the cervix of a woman who has been pregnant and given birth loses its elasticity, making it difficult for a cervical cap to fit properly.

Cervical caps also require spermicide to stop the sperms from entering the uterus. Taking care of a cervical cap is easy and similar to that of a diaphragm, by washing with warm water and soap. However, unlike a diaphragm, a cervical cap can be kept inside for more than 48 hours before sex, so it gives you the chance to be spontaneous during a longer period of time.

Side Effects:

- Vaginal irritation and infection are common side effects of cervical caps.
- These caps are not recommended for women who have been pregnant and gone through a vaginal birth.
- Pregnancy is a possibility for the early months of fitting a cervical cap for the first time.
- Cervical caps are not recommended for women who have a history of Toxic Shock Syndrome, which is a rare but fatal bacterial infection.
- The use of cervical cap rules out the chance of oral sex, because both the odor and the taste of spermicide are appalling.

The effectiveness of a cervical cap depends on its fitting. If fitted correctly, it can prove to be adequately effective against pregnancies, given that you haven't been pregnant before, given birth or suddenly lost/gained significant weight.

Sponge

Sponges work the same way as a cervical cap or diaphragm, by blocking the entrance to the cervix and stopping sperms from entering the uterus. Sponges are small pieces of round foam, made with soft polyurethane with a miniature dent on one side. A thin nylon loop is attached in one side, something like a shoelace. They contain sufficient amount of spermicide that kills sperms and stops conception during and after sex.

Before use, you will need to wet the cervical sponge a little and then insert it into your vagina, all the way up to the opening of your cervix. This can be done as early as 24 hours before having sex, and need to be kept inside at least 8 hours after intercourse. You can have intercourse as many times as you want during this period. Also, it is important to make sure that the sponge completely covers the cervix for the procedure to be effective.

Side Effects:

- As with other barrier methods, the use of sponge rules out oral sex because of the taste and odor of the spermicide.
- Genital irritation is common for cervical sponge.
- Inserting and removing can be a messy process the first few times.

For women who have already had children, the rate of effectiveness is around 80%, which is not a very remarkable number. For other women, if used correctly, the rate of unintentional pregnancy is lower than 9%.

Male and Female condoms

Condoms – both male and female ones – are probably the most popular methods of birth control used around the world. This is because condoms are not only used for birth control, but also as prevention against STDs/STIs. We'll talk more about condoms in the next segment of the book which focuses on safe sex, because condoms are more effective against diseases and infections than just for pregnancies.

Barrier methods are perfect for couples who don't want to risk their fertility with hormonal methods, or for people who prefers temporary solutions to permanent or long-term methods. For women who are sexually active but not regular in their sex life, barrier methods are more preferable to any other procedures.

Emergency Contraceptive Pills

Emergency Contraceptive pills come in handy after you have unprotected sex by mistake or when other birth control methods fail, i.e. condom breaking, diaphragms and cervical caps coming off, etc. If you have had unprotected and spontaneous sex but don't want to conceive, emergency contraceptive pills are what you need!

Emergency Contraceptive Pills (ECP) are more generally known as "morning after pills" but they can be taken up to 72 hours after unprotected sex. However, these pills should only be taken in emergency situations, and not as a regular birth control method.

Usage of these pills depends on the brand you have chosen or the one that is available near you. Some of these pills need to be taken after 12-24 hours of unprotected sex, while others can be taken at any point within 72 hours. Some brands have 2 pills to be taken consecutively one after another; others consist of a single pill to be taken within 3 days (72 hours).

Emergency contraceptive pills only work to delay ovulation and prevent pregnancy, not end one. If a woman becomes pregnant after unprotected sex, taking a pill won't end the pregnancy. The main feat of these pills is to delay the fertilization of the egg until the sperms of your male partner stop being alive and active inside your body. If the egg has already been fertilized by the sperm, the pill won't work. At the same time, it doesn't affect your body or your impending pregnancy.

Emergency Contraceptive Pills (ECP) are known to be 98% effective in women of average weight, i.e. women who weigh less than 154lb (70 kg). A single dose of ECP is good enough for one round of unprotected sex, not for future sexual intercourse in the same cycle

Side Effects:

- Some women complain of headaches, nausea or dizziness after taking a pill. Taking the pill with food usually lessen these side effects.

- Vomiting may occur after taking an emergency contraceptive pill; if you vomit within 2 hours of taking a pill, you need to take another one.

- A number of women complain of symptoms similar to those of period, i.e. abdominal pain, cramps, sore breasts, etc.

It is important to remember that Emergency Contraceptive Pills are not abortion pills. These pills only need to be taken to prevent conception, not to end one. If you are already pregnant, taking a pill will not harm you or your pregnancy in any way.

Fertility Awareness

Being aware of your fertility window and having intercourse accordingly is considered as "natural family planning". This is also known as "Fertility Awareness Method (FAM)" or "Rhythm Method" and based on your own menstrual cycle and body signs.

Following FAM is to restrain from sexual intercourse when you are in the middle of your fertile days. A woman's body goes through change twice during the course of a month – once when she is about to have her period, and again when her body is fertile and ready for conception.

Ovulation in a woman occurs in the middle of her menstrual cycle; most accurately, 14 days before period starts. A single egg is released during this time every month, and that egg lives up to 24 hours inside the body, ready to be fertilized. Sperms that travel from the male partner's body can live inside the female body for as long as 6 days, active and ready to fertilize the egg released in the uterus.

By acute calculations, a total of eight days (six days before ovulation and two days afterwards) in the middle of the menstrual cycle are a woman's fertile days. If you have a fairly regular menstrual cycle, this one week – plus, one more day – in the middle is your fertile period. If you are trying to avoid conception but have unprotected sex, this is the time you need to restrain yourself. By the same logic, couples who are willing to conceive, plan their sexual intercourse during this time to increase their chances of getting pregnant.

This is a highly risky method to follow, with an effectiveness rate of only 75%. This means that if 100 women try to avoid conception via Fertility Awareness Method, 25 of them are likely to get pregnant unintentionally. The rate of conception increases if the woman in question has an irregular menstrual cycle but is healthy and active with an average build.

There are a number of ways to keep track of your ovulation days. First of all, a Calendar-Based Method[5], but this is only possible if you have a regular menstrual cycle. The eight (ten, to be absolutely safe) days in the middle of the menstrual cycle are your fertile days, and should be considered as your days of abstinence if you want to have unprotected sex. The same information is important to men and women who are, in fact, trying to get pregnant.

Another method is the knowledge-based method, which takes into account a number of changes that occur in a woman's body during ovulation. This includes Basal Body Temperature (BBT)[6] which increases during ovulation and Ovulation (Mucus) Method[7] because vaginal discharge also changes and become slippery.

A Sympto-Thermal Method is one which considered all of these methods as well as other physical changes, i.e. soreness of breasts, light spotting, mild abdominal pain or cramps, etc beside basal body temperature and changes in mucus.

Fertility Awareness Method is popular among couples who have religious concerns about birth control, but do not want to conceive. Other than that, this is a risky method to adopt because a woman's menstrual cycle is not always regular and subject to change for a number of reasons.

Side Effects:

- There are no side effects of this method other than the risk of pregnancy because this is not a very effective procedure to follow.

- It is not possible to be spontaneous when using this method, because both partners need to restrain themselves from vaginal intercourse for eight to ten days every month.

- The Fertility Awareness Method requires absolute understanding and commitment from both partners.

- This method is only for preventing pregnancy; unprotected sex can be the cause behind Sexually Transmitted Diseases and Infections when practiced by strangers or people with multiple partners.

In this age where so many methods of birth control are available, Fertility Awareness Method (FAM) is a risky one to adopt, and not completely safe. Besides, it is a lot of work that a woman needs to do – checking for physical changes, keeping a tab on their menstrual cycle, taking regular temperature, etc.

On the other hand, for those preferring this method, there are a lot of phone apps today that can be downloaded to your smartphone and can help ease the trouble of counting and keeping tab the menstrual cycle.

Withdrawal Method for Men

This method is also known as the "Pulling-Out Method" or "Coitus Interruptus". This can be considered an easy method but only if the man is fully aware and in control of his own body, and alert to its needs – which can be hard during passionate intercourse.

Withdrawal Method is when the male partner pulls out his penis out of the women's vagina just before he ejaculates so that his semen does not enter the woman's body. It is rightly one of the oldest methods of birth control of the world, discovered way before any other methods of birth control had been invented.

Pulling-Out Method comes in handy when sex is spontaneous and there isn't any form of birth control method available around, or when the woman isn't using birth control methods but doesn't want to conceive. It only works if the man in question successfully manages to pull out his genitalia right before he ejaculates; if even a little semen enters the woman, pregnancy can happen.

Withdrawal Method is free, easy and convenient, but it is not always effective. In moments of passion, it becomes hard for a man to stay alert enough to withdraw when he needs to, and ends up ejaculating inside the woman's vagina. This method is completely in a man's control; a woman has nothing to do but to remind her partner to pull out before ejaculation.

Side Effects:

- This is not a method many men prefer; it interrupts sexual pleasure because they have to keep alert at all times and this can disrupt their enjoyment during sex.

- Withdrawal method is a messy procedure. The man has to ejaculate outside the vagina, which could mean anywhere ranging from the woman's body to the bed, the floor or on clothes – a mess to clean up later.

- Easy as it might seem, this is an unreliable method that most physicians don't recommend.

- Most importantly, this is not a scientific method that can ensure birth control. Pregnancy is still possible if a man pulls out in the nick of time because there are some sperm present in the pre-cum or the pre-ejaculation that can enter the woman's vagina.

Pulling-Out method decreases the fun of sex for most men, and this is not a method they are a fan of. Besides, this method is completely under the control of the male partner; if they are not very caring of their partner's desire to not get pregnant, matters can get out of hand. In cases where alternative birth control methods are not present, withdrawal method followed by emergency contraceptive pills can ensure no conception.

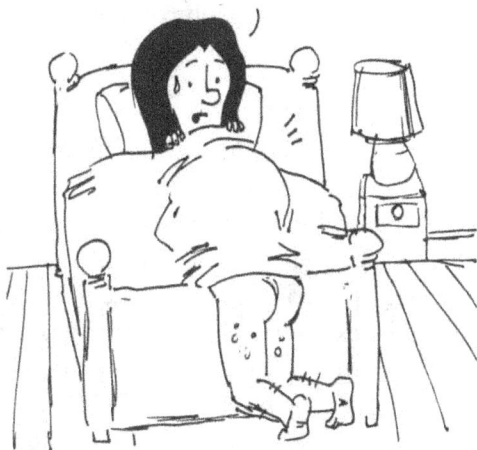

Choosing the Right Birth Control Method

For different couples, the requirements for birth control are different. While some couples prefer to be spontaneous in their romance, others prefer an effective solution. While a few couples choose for a permanent solution because they already have the perfect number of children they want, others prefer to keep their options open.

Your choice of birth control depends on your lifestyle and your preference.

SPONTANEITY

If you want your sex life to be spontaneous and have no immediate plans to have children, a long-term birth control method is what you need. An Implant or Intra-Uterine Device (IUD) inserted into the woman's body will provide the couple the chance of 3 to 12 years of unprotected sex with no worries of pregnancies. Besides making your love life spontaneous, these methods also happen to be up to 99% effective, which means that only 1 woman in 100 is likely to become pregnant while using one of these long-term methods.

Of the three different methods of long-term birth control, - Implant and Hormonal and Copper IUD - it is the use of Copper IUD which is the most effective and gives the longest protection against unintentional pregnancy. According to a study[8] published online on August 2010 by Bliss Kaneshiro and Tod Aeby in the International Journal of Women's Health, this method is used by more than 150 million women all around the world with less than 1% failure rate.

COST

When it comes to cost, there are several ways to look at the different methods of birth control: *cost per unit and overall cost*. For example, an IUD insertion may cost hundreds of dollars the first time, but each insertion lasts for years; especially, a copper IUD lasts for more than 10/12 years, which significantly decreases the cost endured per year.

In the same way, a pack of condoms – each containing 3 to 4 units – costs about a dollar or so, depending on the brand. It is really up to the couple how often they have intercourse and how many packets they need per day or week. Even if this is a couple who has intercourse fairly often, i.e. 300 times a year while the average 3-pack condom packet costs $1, that's $100 per year.

In the United States, insertion of an IUD costs around $210 to $800 for someone who isn't covered by insurance. This may sound like a lot of money, but remember: *a single insertion lasts years*. A pack of condoms may only cost a dollar, but if you are sexually active throughout the year, the total cost isn't that low. Therefore, a lot depends on the fact whether you are covered by insurance or if you are willing to spend a lot of money at one time, or over a period of time.

PERMANENCE

If it is a permanent solution you are looking for, nothing is better than a male vasectomy or a female sterilization. These two methods are 100% effective as well as permanent and cannot be reversed. Only people who are completely sure they already have the children they desire or don't want any more biological children should go through these methods to enjoy worry-free sex with their partner for the rest of their lives.

Although reversal is possible in some cases, the results aren't very impressive, especially when considered after more than 10 years of the original surgery. According to a study[9] published on October 2012 by Aaron n M. Bernie, Charles Osterberg, Peter J. Stahl Ranjith Ramasamy and Marc Goldstein, a reversal in vasectomy – a rather demanding and difficult procedure – results in pregnancy in around 40%-80% of the cases, depending on age and circumstances.

RECURRING MEDICAL INTERVENTION

For some methods, regular (almost) trips to the doctor is necessary, *i.e. a birth control shot.* Although this method is about 94% effective, going to the doctor for a shot every 3 months could be a bother many women prefer not to go through. Besides, some other barrier methods – namely, a vaginal ring, cap, sponge or a diaphragm – can sometimes get stuck within the vagina which could mean a trip to the doctor as well.

If you want a birth control method that you can just have and be done with without having to worry too much about, long-term solutions like an implant or an IUD is the best solution for you. Once inserted, you can carry on for 3 years (for an implant) or 10/12 years (for copper IUD) without having to think about birth control ever again.

ANNOYING SIDE EFFECTS

Side effects of some of the birth control methods are annoying, especially the symptoms that are similar to those of pregnancy like dizziness, soreness of breasts, nausea, abdominal pain, etc. Methods that increase the chance of too much side effects are hormonal contraceptives like pills, injections, patches and rings. Barrier methods also have some side effects that could make a woman decide to switch methods and try something else.

The methods with the least number of side effects are probably the simplest ones – fertility awareness in women and withdrawal method in men. Since these are natural methods that require nothing, there are no side effects or symptoms to worry about. However, since they are also unreliable methods, the next best thing would be to rely on long term solutions like an implant or IUD. The side effects of these methods may be prominent at first but slowly fade away over months.

EFFECTIVENESS

When it comes to effectiveness, the two methods that are most effective are vasectomy and female tubal ligation. However, these are not methods that many people would choose, especially young people who have the desire for biological children in the future. They prefer the use of long-time methods, hormonal methods and barriers to prevent pregnancy in the present but keep their options open for the future.

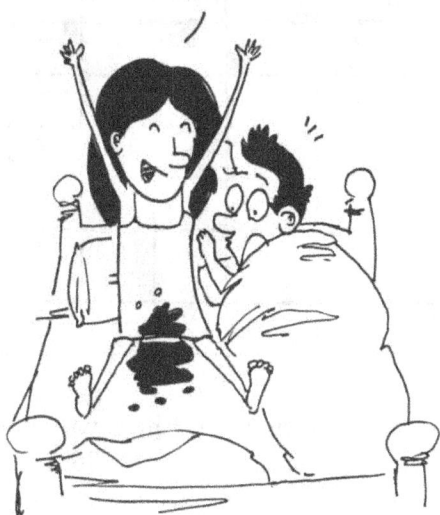

In a nutshell

COMPARE	Permanent Method	Long-term Method	Hormonal Method	Barrier Method	Withdrawal Method	Fertility Awareness	Emergency Contraceptive Pill
Spontaneity	√	√	√	×	√	×	√
Inexpensive	×	×	×	√	√	√	√
Permanence	√	×	×	×	×	×	×
Side Effects	×	×	√	√	×	×	√
Medical Intervention	×	×	√	√	×	×	×
Effectiveness	√	√	√	√	×	×	√

This table, hopefully, will help you choose a birth control method that fits your lifestyle and your requirements. If you can't decide, why not just pick the one that seems logical and try it? If you face any kind of problems, you can switch methods.

The Need for Safe Sex

Unprotected sex is usually fine when it is with a partner or a spouse, but not for those with multiple partners. When engaging in unprotected intercourse with someone who might have multiple partners, or when you enjoy sex with multiple partners, you increase the risk of something more than pregnancy.

An unintentional pregnancy is only one of the worries to have after unprotected intercourse with someone you are not too familiar with or know much about. Emergency Contraceptive Pills can be taken if you are worried about a conception after spending unprotected time with a new partner, but what you can't save yourself against are Sexually Transmitted Diseases (STDs) and Infections (STIs).

What are Sexually Transmitted Diseases (STDs)?

These are diseases that pass from one person to another through unprotected sexual acts. Infections that people carry in their body are passed on to others through sex, and these infections are caused by parasites, yeast, virus and bacteria.

STDs are common for both genders, but more serious in women, especially if they are pregnant. If an expecting mother comes in sexual contact with another person who has STD, it could mean grave danger for the unborn child.

What are Sexually Transmitted Infections (STIs)?

All kinds of Sexually Transmitted Diseases (STDs) start off as infections due to coming in contact with an infected person. When someone has an STI, it simply means they have an infection passed on to them by someone else; their infection hasn't developed into a full-fledged disease yet. In other words, Sexually Transmitted Infections (STIs) are a less negative version of a STD, used mainly to remove the stigma behind the concept.

When an infected person isn't aware of any symptoms or hasn't developed a disease, it is a STI. On the other hand, when symptoms flourish and the infection take the form of a disease, it can be said that the person in question has a Sexually Transmitted Disease (STD). For example, HIV is a virus that a person can carry in their body and not even be aware of any discomfort. HIV is a virus, and thus, an infection – STI. When that virus turns into AIDS, which is a disease grown from the virus, it becomes a disease and the person is said to have a STD.

In the same way, a woman can carry the Human Papilloma Virus (HPV) but not have any symptoms of the virus at all; she has an STI. If the same virus develops into cervical cancer, which is definitely a disease – she will have STD, a disease transmitted through sexual contract.

Therefore, all STDs start off as infections, but with treatment, not all infections may develop into full-fledged diseases. Infections that are caused by bacteria, yeast or parasites can be quite easily cured by medication and treatment; it is the infections caused by virus that are deadlier and harder to cure!

Different kinds of STIs and STDs

There are over 20 different types of Sexually Transmitted Infections and Diseases out there, and they can be divided into three different categories:

- Those which clears on its own over time;
- Those which are curable with the correct treatments; and
- Those which don't have a cure yet.

Infections that Clear Over Time

Some kinds of infections clear on its own in a healthy person without much need for treatment or medications. These are usually caused by skin-to-skin contract with an infected person or during sexual intercourse, and can be seen in both men and women.

Human Papilloma Virus (HPV)

There are some forms of HPV that stays dormant in the human body and goes away on its own within 2 to 4 years. They usually stay dormant in the body but can spread to an uninfected person through sexual contact. Some HPV infections can lead to genital warts, which may need treatment to go away. In most cases, these infections are cured in a few months; in some rare cases, HPV infections can take up to 4 years to disappear.

Molluscum Contagiosum (MC)

These are a special form of viruses that go away on its own after 6 to 18 months. This virus surfaces as small but firm spots on the skin that are itchy but not painful. Despite their look, these are rather harmless infections that don't need any specific treatment to go away.

Hepatitis A Virus (HAV)

Hepatitis A Virus can be controlled with immunization, but it is not a harmful infection when contracted. This virus can live inside the body for 5/6 months and then go away on its own without any treatment.

Acute Hepatitis B Virus (HBV)

This is another quite harmless virus that can live in the body for six months, and then clear away. No treatment is needed for acute Hepatitis B Virus.

Acute Hepatitis C Virus (HCV)

In 1 out of 5 cases, acute Hepatitis C Virus clears on its own without any treatment. In other severe cases, this virus can lead to chronic infection which needs to be treated intensively.

Infections that Need to be Treated

People who are sexually active with multiple partners come in contact with Sexually Transmitted Infections (STIs) at least once in their lives. This could be a simple infection that can be cured by a single dose of antibiotics, like Chlamydia and Gonorrhea; or, it could be an infection like Syphilis that needs treatment in a number of stages.

Gonorrhea

Gonorrhea is better known as "The Clap" or "The Drip", and is spread through vaginal, anal or oral sex, or via sex toys that haven't been cleaned properly. This is one of the most common infections to come into contact in the United States of America, with more than 333,004 cases reported in 2013, according to the Center for Disease Control.[10] *[Source]* However, since most of the infected men and women do not get any symptoms of this infection, the actual number is definitely much higher than the ones reported.

Gonorrhea usually affects the rectum, cervix or urethra; or the throat, in case of transmission through oral sex. The number of women infected from this bacterium is more than men, and the younger generation aged 15-29 are affected more. Antibiotics and abstinence from intercourse for a few weeks can cure gonorrhea completely.

Chlamydia

It is an infection caused by the bacteria *Chlamydia Trachomatis* and is spread via anal, oral and vaginal sex as well as sex toys. Chlamydia can occur in both men and women and has very few symptoms in the infected person. Getting tested for Chlamydia is a good way to keep this infection in check.

It is relatively easy to treat Chlamydia if diagnosed early, with a single dose of antibiotics. If not diagnosed and left untreated, it can lead to infertility in women; if pregnant women comes in sexual contact with an infected person, the baby could be born with the infection. Infants and children who contract the infection can become blind or get pneumonia.

Scabies

Scabies is a special kind of infection where tiny insect-like mites crawl under the skin of the infected person and lay eggs; even staying neat and clean all the time cannot save a person from this infection if they come in contact with an infected person.

Scabies spreads through personal and sexual contact as well as skin-to-skin contact in very crowded places. It is more prominent and common in children than in adults and can be treated with special creams and lotions. Besides, it is important to minimize skin-to-skin contact with the infected person and to vigorously clean all their clothes, bedding and towels to stop this infection from spreading.

Syphilis

Caused by bacteria named *spirochete,* Syphilis is one of the oldest and most common sexually transmitted infections known to man. Syphilis is contacted through anal, oral and vaginal sex, and even by kissing or intimately touching an infected person. Common symptoms of this infection include more than one painful ulcer, soreness in the throat, rashes, pain in the joints and tiredness.

Unlike other infections, Syphilis attacks in different stages; the different stages have different symptoms, side effects as well as treatments. In the initial and secondary stages, penicillin can be effective in curing primary Syphilis. High dosage of antibiotics may be needed in the later stages, and cure can be almost impossible in the last stages.

Trichomoniasis

Trichomoniasis is also known as a "trich" and caused by a parasite called *trichomonas vaginalis*. This infection is extremely common in developing countries, with more than 3.7 million infected people in the United States of America, according to the Center for Disease Control.[11] [Source]

"Trich" is usually spread through sexual contact between an infected person and an uninfected person – which can be between a man and a woman, or two people of the same sex. In women, the vagina, vulva and urethra are infected the most and in men, the inside of the penis. A single dosage of antibiotic is enough to cure Trichomoniasis if diagnosed at the right time.

Pubic Lice/Crabs

This is not really an infection but small lice-like insects that settle in a person's pubic hair where they settle and lay eggs. This infestation spreads when an unaffected person comes into skin-to-skin contact with an infected person in the pubic regions.

Itchy genitals are one of the most common symptoms of pubic lice, or "Crabs" – as they are more generally known as. Special lotions, creams and shampoo are available for removal of pubic lice which are very effective.

Infections that Have No Cure Yet

Infections that are incurable are the ones that gradually turn into diseases. While some of these diseases are treatable while not curable, some are actually fatal. It is the dangerous and fatal diseases, like AIDS, that we should be careful about when we are enjoying intercourse with partners we are not committed to, or we are not much familiar with.

Human Immuno-Deficiency Virus/Acquired Immune Deficiency Syndrome (HIV/AIDS)

HIV/AIDS is probably the worst Sexually Transmitted Diseases (STD) to date, one that has no cure and no definite treatment yet. HIV is a chronic infection which leads to AIDS if not diagnosed and treated immediately. HIV attacks the immune system in our body, and AIDS makes it hard for the body to fight off any other diseases and infections, something as simple as a cold or the flu.

Since its discovery first in the 1980s, the casualty of AIDS has reached more than 35 million all over the world. In the United States of America alone, more than 39,513 people were diagnosed with this disease in the year 2015, according to the Center for Disease Control. It is the gays and the bisexuals, particularly men, who are more effected than other people throughout the world; they account for 82% of all the men diagnosed everywhere.[12] [Source]

Every year, millions of dollars are being funded for research into curing HIV/AIDS, not just in USA but all over the world. With the advancements of medical science, people affected with AIDS are living a much longer and healthier life than before. However, there are still no definite cure of AIDS as of yet, which makes this one of the deadliest STDs of the world.

Oral/Genital Herpes

Two different types of viruses HSV-1 and HSV-2 are responsible for oral and genital herpes respectively. Both of these herpes are spread via sexual intercourse with an infected person – oral, anal or vaginal sex, as well as kissing or sharing a spoon. The initial symptoms of Oral and Genital Herpes are similar to flu, including body ache, swollen lymphs and fever.

It is possible for an individual to be affected by both types of herpes at the same time; actually, in more than half the cases, oral herpes slowly leads to genital herpes in an infected person. There are some medications that can reduce the frequency and the severity of herpes, as well as stop genital herpes from spreading to an unaffected partner. Other than that, there is unfortunately no permanent cure of Oral/Genital Herpes yet.

Human Papilloma Virus (HPV)

There are some strains of HPV which are not curable and cause more permanent damage in a human being. These strains can lead to genital warts or cervical cancer. Cancer caused by HPV is quite common all over the world; in the United States alone, more than 27,000 men and women are diagnosed with HPV cancer, according to CDC.[13] *[Source]*

There are some vaccines available now that can prevent the growth of genital warts in men and women. Before these vaccines were invented, around 360,000 people were diagnosed with genital warts every year in the United States. At any point in time, 1 in every 100 people were affected with this infection, according to CDC.[14] *[Source]*

There are some HPV that clears away in a human body on its own; in other cases, the body becomes susceptible to genital warts and cervical cancer which regrettably, is more serious and doesn't have a cure yet.

Chronic Hepatitis B & C Virus (HBV & HCV)

HBV and HCV virus attacks and impairs the liver in the human body, and often damages it beyond repair. Chronic Hepatitis can be diagnosed within a few months of being affected with the Hepatitis B or C virus, and these viruses continue to live inside the human body for the rest of that person's life.

Hepatitis B Virus is spread through sexual contact, as well as from mother to child through childbirth. This disease is more deadly for infants, with a staggering rate of 90% of them becoming chronically infected. There are some vaccines available for HBV but they are not always completely effective.[15] *[Source]*

Sexual intercourse with an HCV-infected person can spread this virus to an uninfected person, as well as an infected mother giving birth. Of all the people infected with this disease, 15% to 25% of them are lucky enough to clear away without any treatment or medication. However, for the rest of the population, Hepatitis C Virus (HCV) becomes chronic and needs to be carried inside the body for the rest of their lives.

There is currently no vaccine available for HCV, unfortunately, but research is going on in this sector for a number of years.

The best way to deal with Sexually Transmitted Infections (STIs) and Diseases (STDs) are not through treatment or medication, but by preventing them. Sex needs to be safe for us to enjoy it completely and without worries, and the best and most effective ways to enjoy worry-free sexual intercourse are explained in details in the next chapter of this book.

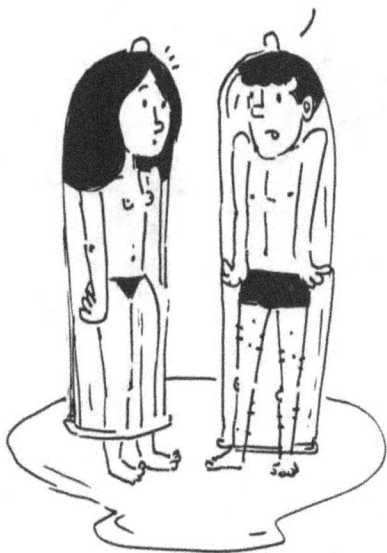

Well, these were the larger
ones... I think now we're safe.

Live Safe with Safe Sex

Birth control and safe sex are two completely different concepts, although both related to sexual intercourse. With birth control methods, you are only preventing conception; whereas, having safe sex saves you from Sexually Transmitted Diseases (STDs) and Infections (STIs).

Safe sex is a much varied concept of sexual intercourse. Only vaginal sexual intercourse between a fertile man and a woman can result in a pregnancy, which is easy to prevent with more than 20 different methods to choose from. Unsafe sex, on the other hand, can occur between people of all genders – between a man and a woman, as well as between two and more people of the same gender. It is not only vaginal sex that can result in transmission of STDs and STIs, but oral and anal sex, as well as skin-to-skin contact.

One infected person with multiple partners can transmit their infections to a number of people who, in turn, spreads the infection further. This is how these infections spread across the population – from infected people practicing unsafe and unprotected sexual intercourse with multiple partners. The best way to prevent STDs and STIs from spreading is of course, to practice safe sex, but at the same time, to stay informed and updated.

Awareness and Knowledge

Get Tested As Often As Possible

It is important that you get tested and stay updated with your own body at all times. There are a lot of STIs out there that have no symptoms, such as Chlamydia and Gonorrhea, and are not easy to diagnose by oneself. Left untreated, these infections could lead to serious problems and often cause infertility in women.

Some Sexually Transmitted Infections (STIs) are harder to diagnose because their symptoms are similar to flu or other similar illnesses, like Syphilis. The symptoms of these infections are often misdiagnosed or even avoided, which may lead to more severe diseases in the future, if not treated immediately.

The best way to avoid such situations is to get tested as often as possible, especially if you have an active sexual life and multiple partners. A simple visit to your physician, gynecologist or the local STD Testing center will give you all the information you need – for both men and women. People of both genders, regardless of how much sexual intercourse they enjoy, should get themselves tested often, especially women if they are thinking of having children in the near future or have an infant they care for. Even people who have single partners and are in a committed relationship should visit a STD Testing Center sometimes because there are many other ways that these infections spread other than direct sexual intercourse.

Get Vaccinated

Vaccinations are available for some STIs, namely HAV, HBV and HPV; research is going on to develop both the prevention and vaccines for other common STIs. It is important that you, and the people you are having sex with, are updated and vaccinated for you to enjoy safe sex.

According to the Center for Disease Control, the HPV Vaccination should be mandatory for every female from ages 9 to 26, and for boys from ages 11 to 21. This is especially important for men who are likely to have intercourse with other men, i.e. gays and bisexuals.[16] *[Source]*

Know Your Own Body, and Your Partner's

Symptoms of most STIs are easy to miss and can be misdiagnosed with rashes, flu, allergies and other similar illnesses. For example, symptoms of Syphilis include a sore throat, tiredness and rashes; at the same time, symptoms of Gonorrhea include painful urinating in men and women, as well as abnormal vaginal discharge and heavier spotting in women. It is very easy to dismiss these slight symptoms as normal, especially if we are not familiar with our own bodies and that of our partner's.

At the first sign of such abnormalities of any kind, a visit to the doctor is most crucial. Visiting your doctor, preferably with your partner, to discuss the symptoms will help you understand if you have contacted any STIs that need to be treated.

Get Treated As Soon As Possible

Treatment for most Sexually Transmitted Infections (STIs) is easy and speedy. Consulting a doctor and taking the right dosage of antibiotics can help cure these infections almost immediately. Most of the common STIs - namely Gonorrhea, Syphilis and Chlamydia - need only one dose of antibiotics to go away.

However, these infections need to be treated as soon as they are diagnosed. If left untreated, seemingly harmless infections can lead to diseases and serious conditions later.

When diagnosed with an infection, it is also important that you contact all the partners you have enjoyed sexual contact with recently so that they can get themselves tested as well. If you are in a committed relationship with someone, taking your partner for testing and treatment is also important for your full recovery.

Behave Responsibly

Be Honest About Your History

If you are engaging in sexual contact with someone new, it is always important to be honest about your sexual and health history and ask the same of your partner. If you have recently been diagnosed with a Sexually Transmitted Infection (STI) and undergoing treatment, be honest about it before you start anything. If you are honest about yourself, it will encourage your new partner to be honest about their sexual history as well.

Choose a Single Partner to Commit To

One of the best ways to avoid STIs is to stay in a committed relationship with a single partner. Since these infections mainly spread because of sexual contact with multiple partners, staying in a monogamous relationship decreases the risk of contracting STIs. In a fair and loving monogamous relationship, both partners are loyal to each other and have sexual contact only with each other, thus not bring any unwanted virus or germs into the equation.

If it is monogamy that you are choosing, be sure that the relationship is mutually monogamous, i.e. both partners are willing to have sexual contact with each other only and no one else. This includes any kind of sexual contact, including kissing and intimate touching as they too can increase chances of some infection.

Explore Alternate Methods of Sex

Although not so satisfying, there are other methods of sex that you can explore that doesn't require anal, oral or vaginal sex, or even intimate touching. Masturbation or mutual masturbation, sexting or talking about sex, cyber sex or phone sex - these are all alternative methods of sex that can bring two people closer to each other.

If you are in a new relationship with someone you are not yet sure of, these alternative methods of sex are better than direct intercourse until you can be honest about each other's history. Although these methods are not as satisfying as sex, they are safe and useful in getting to know each other. If you want some physical contact with each other, you can also try kissing, massaging or fondling as foreplay but not end up having sexual intercourse before you are ready.

Many men and women out there prefer not to engage in sexual intercourse immediately after meeting someone new, for personal reasons as well as for safety purposes. These alternate methods would be perfect for them to try.

Don't Mix Sex with Drugs and Alcohol

Taking drugs or consuming alcohol doesn't only lower your inhibitions, they impact your ability to think rationally. Under the influence of drugs and alcohol, you are more likely to do something you wouldn't do under normal circumstances, such as have unprotected sexual intercourse with a stranger. Actions like these don't only increase your chances of unintentional pregnancy, but of contracting STIs as well.

Besides, under the influence of drugs and alcohol, you might automatically turn into a consenting adult whereas you had no intention of having sex with someone. This is especially true in case of women; they often find themselves in compromising situations and under attack with no recollection of anything that had happened previously. Therefore, if there is a chance of drinking excessively at a gathering/party or using drugs, it is better to have someone trusted and responsible around to keep an eye on you.

Using the Correct Protection

Using Male Condoms

Male condoms are probably the most widely used method of protection all around the world, both for birth control and for protection against STIs. Condoms are easily available anywhere and inexpensive; often, they are available free in hospitals, clinics and locations that support Planned Parenthood Programs.

Condoms are made from latex; for people who are allergic to latex, condoms made of polyurethane are also available. They are male contraceptives that need to be worn on the penis of the male partner just before penetration. For extra safety against Sexually Transmitted Infections (STIs), condoms should be used before anal and oral sex besides vaginal sex. Contrary to popular belief, specially-ribbed and extra-thin condoms are actually responsible for heightening pleasure during intercourse and making sex more enjoyable. They do not cause hindrance in the middle of sexual intercourse in any way; rather, the act of putting on a male condom is sometimes considered an important part of foreplay.

When used correctly, condoms rarely tear or rip-off. If that happens during sex, it is important that the female partner take an emergency contraceptive pill to reduce the chances of pregnancy; if it is STI that both partners are worried about, testing themselves within 10 days of unprotected sex should be enough.

Male condoms are compact and lightweight, and can be carried anywhere in a pocket or inside a purse. If you are sexually active – with or without a committed partner – stocking up on condoms is a good idea for both men and women. Male condoms don't just protect the women against an unintentional pregnancy, but both partners from different kinds of infections. All types of couples – heterosexual and bisexuals, as well as gays – should consider the use of condoms before engaging in sexual contact.

According to the Center for Disease Control, condoms don't only protect us from contacting the Human Immunodeficiency Virus that leads to AIDS but other infections that are caused by exchanging of genital fluid, i.e. Chlamydia, Trichomoniasis, Gonorrhea and sometimes, genital herpes. [17][Source] This is the reason male condoms are a preferred choice of protection of a large portion of the population all over the world.

Female Condoms

Female condoms follow the same mechanism as a male condom, but they are for the use of the female partner as opposed to the male. Before intercourse, female condoms need to be inserted inside the vagina up to the cervix where they would trap the sperm ejaculated by the male penis. After each use, a female condom needs to be removed and thrown away; they are not to be reused a second time.

Success rate of female condoms are only 79%, which makes them a risky method to choose for birth control. This particular method is more preferably considered to provide protection against HIV as well as other similar infections.

Correctly inserting a female condom may require practice; they are trickier than putting on a male condom and have the chance of loosening and disappearing inside the vagina. It is important that you do not use a male and a female condom at the same time. Doing so will create friction inside the vagina, resulting in tear and ripping. For birth control, combining female condoms with any other birth control method is a good idea.

Dental Dams

Dental dams are important protection against infections for oral sex. They are latex sheets, square in size that need to be wrapped around the penis or the female genital during oral sex. They prevent bodily fluids, genitalia fluids and blood to enter the mouth and cause infection.

Using dental dams correctly can keep a person safe from infections that occur due to skin-to-skin contact in sensitive areas, and needs to be discarded immediately after use. They are available in affordable prices in most drug stores and clinics; in absence of one, a regular male or female condom can be cut open and cleaned to be used as a dental dam.

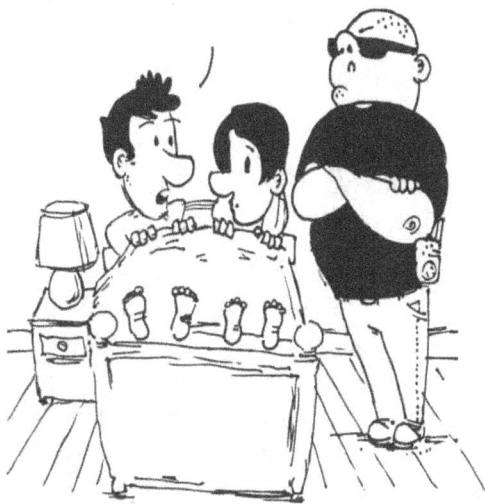

Last Words

All these information about birth control and safe sex does not decrease the pleasure of sex in any way. Rather, when you are safe from unintentional pregnancy and Sexually Transmitted Diseases (STDs), you can immerse yourself in enjoying sex without a care in this world.

Whether you are having intercourse with your spouse, a long-time partner or someone new, it is important to always be cautious – regarding an accidental conception, or contacting an infection that can prove to be dangerous for both of you in the future. The best way to be sure of that not happening is to be aware and updated, and to choose the perfect method that suits your lifestyle and your preference – both for birth control and for prevention against STDs.

This book is a complete guideline to everything you need to know about both these techniques. It has everything every sexually active man and woman needs to know about sex, and save themselves from a weary future. Newer and better methods of birth control and safe sex are emerging to make our sex lives better and more exciting, and it is important that we keep ourselves updated with them.

I wish you a happy and safe sex life!

Glossary

(In Order of Appearance)

Sexually Active - This term refers to a person who has sexual intercourse regularly, with a single partner or multiple partners.

Birth Control - Birth control is a method or a device to prevent pregnancy chosen by a man or a woman who is sexually active.[Source]

Childbearing Age - The age range when a woman is capable of getting pregnant and giving birth. [Source]

Safe Sex - The act of sexual intercourse when both (or more) parties have taken special precaution so that they don't conceive or contract Sexually Transmitted Diseases from an infected person. [Source]

Sexually Transmitted Diseases (STDs) - Diseases that spread from an infected person to an uninfected one, via oral, anal and vaginal sex as well as through unclean sex toys, kissing or intimate touching. [Source]

Sperms - Reproductive cells in human beings that cause conception; they are only present in male partners and are transferred to the female partner via vaginal intercourse. [Source]

Semen - Semen are organic fluids that contain sperms and are only present in male partners. [Source]

Scrotum - A scrotum is a male physical structure that is one of the main components of the male reproductive system, important for sexual intercourse. [Source]

Masturbation - Is the act of stimulating one's own genitals for sexual pleasure until the act leads to an orgasm, which is the height of sexual pleasure. [Source]

Fallopian Tubes - The Fallopian Tubes are two very fine tubes running from the uterus to the ovaries, which plays an important role in female fertilization and reproduction. [Source]

Ectopic Pregnancy - Abnormal pregnancies when fertilization in a woman occurs somewhere other than the uterus and usually results in a missed abortion. [Source]

Progesterone - Progesterone is a special hormone in the female body that plays a special role in menstruation cycle, reproduction and conception. [Source]

Uterus - Is the main reproductive organ of the female body, where the fetus is developed in pregnancy. The uterus is connected to the Fallopian tubes at one end and opens to the vagina on the other. [Source]

Ovulation - Ovulation is the process of an egg released from the ovaries which happens one every month. [Source]

Vaginal Discharge - This is a mixture of a number of liquids that are present in the vagina, namely cells, liquid, bacteria and lubricants. This liquid is continuously exiting through the vaginal opening, more so in special occasions. [Source]

Oral Sex - The stimulation of one's genitals (men or women) using their partners mouth, lips, teeth or tongue. [Source]

Anal Sex - The sexual intercourse between a man's penis another person's anus, or rectum. [Source]

Fertility Window - The window of fertility is the few days in the middle of a woman's menstrual cycle when she is fertile and capable of conception. [Source]

Rectum - The rectum is the last part of a person's large intestine, ending is an opening at the back of the body between the legs. In homosexual men and heterosexual women, the rectum plays an important part in anal sex. [Source]

Notes

1. Jones, J., Mosher, W., & Daniels, K. (October 2012). Current contraceptive use in the United States, 2006-2010, and changes in patters of use since 1995. *National Health Statistics Report,* No.60. https://www.cdc.gov/nchs/data/nhsr/nhsr060.pdf

2. Center for Disease Control and Prevention. www.cdc.gov

3. Daniels, K., Mosher, W., & Jones, J. (February 2013). Contraceptive methods women have ever used: United States 1982-2010. *National Health Statistics Report,* No.62. https://www.cdc.gov/nchs/data/nhsr/nhsr062.pdf

4. Jones, R.K. & Dreweke, J. (April 2011). Countering conventional wisdom: New evidence on religion and contraceptive use. *Guttmacher Institute.* http://www.thestranger.com/images/blogimages/2011/04/14/1302811453-religion-and-contraceptive-use.pdf

5. Calendar-based methods are various methods of estimating a woman's likelihood of fertility, based on a record of the length of previous menstrual cycles. Various methods are known as the Knaus–Ogino Method and the Rhythm Method. The Standard Days Method is also considered a calendar-based method, because when using it, a woman tracks the days of her menstrual cycle without observing her physical fertility signs. The Standard Days Method is based on a fixed formula taking into consideration the timing of ovulation, the functional life of the sperm and the ovum, and the resulting likelihood of pregnancy on particular days of the menstrual cycle.

6. Your basal body temperature is your temperature when you're fully at rest. Ovulation may cause a slight increase in basal body temperature. You'll be most fertile during the two to three days before your temperature rises. By tracking your basal body temperature each day, you may be able to predict when you'll ovulate. In turn, this may help you determine when you're most likely to conceive.

7. The cervical mucus method is based on careful observation of mucus patterns during the course of your menstrual cycle. Before ovulation, cervical secretions change — creating an environment that helps sperm travel through the cervix, uterus and fallopian tubes to the egg. By recognizing the changing characteristics of your cervical mucus, you can predict when you'll ovulate. In turn, this may help you determine when you're most likely to conceive.

8. Kaneshiro, B. & Aeby, T. (2010). Long-Term safety, efficacy, and patient acceptability of the intrauterine copper T-380A contraceptive devise. *International Journal of Women's Health*, 2, 211-220.

9. Bernie, A.M., Osterberg, E.C., Stahl,P.J., Ramasamy, R., and Goldstein, M. (2012). Vasectomy reversal in humans. *Spermatogenesis*, 2(4).

10. Center for Disease Control and Prevention. *2015 Sexually Transmitted Diseases Surveillance*, https://www.cdc.gov/std/stats15/gonorrhea.htm

11. Center for Disease Control and Prevention. *Trichomoniasis — CDC Fact Sheet*. https://www.cdc.gov/std/trichomonas/STDFact-Trichomoniasis.htm

12. Center for Disease Control and Prevention. *HIV in the United States: At a glance*. https://www.cdc.gov/hiv/statistics/overview/ataglance.html

13. Center for Disease Control and Prevention. *What is HPV?* https://www.cdc.gov/hpv/parents/whatishpv.html

14. Center for Disease Control and Prevention. *Genital HPV Infection – Fact Sheet.* https://www.cdc.gov/std/hpv/stdfact-hpv.htm

15. Center for Disease Control and Prevention. *Viral Hepatitis – Hepatitis B Information.* https://www.cdc.gov/hepatitis/hbv/index.htm

16. Center for Disease Control and Prevention. *Human Papillomavirus (HPV).* https://www.cdc.gov/hpv/parents/questions-answers.html

17. Center for Disease Control and Prevention. *Condom Effectiveness.* https://www.cdc.gov/condomeffectiveness/brief.html

About the Author

Dr. Mary Ann Martínez is a Licensed Professional Counselor, and a Marriage, Family and Sex Therapist. She runs a successful private practice in Puerto Rico, where she has been helping individuals, couples, and families for more than 20 years.

You can contact her at mmartinez@consejeria.net.

Other books by the author:

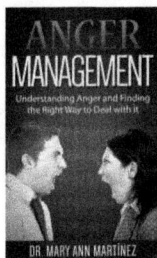

Anger Management: Understanding anger and finding the right way to deal with it .

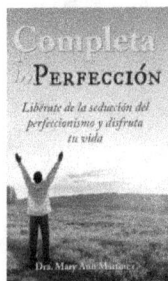

Completa Imperfección: Libérate de la seducción del perfeccionismo y disfruta tu vida.

www.ingramcontent.com/pod-product-compliance
Lightning Source LLC
Chambersburg PA
CBHW050554280326
41933CB00011B/1838